THE COVID-19 VACCINE

An Expert's Medical Guide for All

Zeil Rosenberg, M.D.

Thanks to my wife Ingkan and our children Jenica and Jason, without whose support my life in the world of vaccines would not be possible.

INTRODUCTION

At the time of this writing, the COVID-19 pandemic has led to over 95 million cases and 2.0 million deaths worldwide, with over 23 million cases and 400,000 lives lost in the United States alone. Humankind needs solutions and needs them now. However, we have to trust that these solutions will do the job without any unintended consequences for our health.

Vaccine scientists are seen by many in the scientific community as falling into the category of miracle makers. Salk and Sabin vanquished polio from the US, and now virtually all of the world, with their remarkable and novel vaccines. Public health experts have had their impact, as well. The eradication of smallpox in 1978, with millions of lives spared, was due to better administration of existing smallpox vaccines using a novel, tiny bifurcated needle combined with a ring vaccination strategy that prioritized scarce vaccination program resources and targeted disease hotspots.

In the past, however, some vaccine development and distribution efforts – such as the swine flu vaccine crisis of 1976 -- were embarked upon in anticipation of a pandemic that never materialized. The vaccine was released prematurely without the necessary clinical studies needed to assure complete vaccine safety. These efforts created erosion of the public's trust in government-led vaccine response efforts that persists to this day.

However, the situation today has changed radically. We are enduring a global pandemic, with widespread lockdowns to prevent disease transmission and further deaths, while small businesses, and the hopes and dreams of their owners, are being crushed underfoot.

We are also in a new age, where scientific breakthroughs in the biological sciences can be trained on this new enemy. New, next-generation methods of vaccine design, in addition to improved data-driven systems of vaccine safety monitoring, have made our vaccine supply the safest ever. And vast resources have been allocated to a number of vaccine clinical trials, so that these trials can be completed by multiple vaccine companies in parallel as quickly as possible.

But is it enough? Should we be the first to take these new COVID-19 vaccines, some of which may be designed like no other before them? During a time when the rapid development of a COVID-19 vaccine has been pushed to the limit? Where a vaccine may not be available immediately to all but the most high-risk individuals?

As a trained physician and epidemiologist with decades of experience organizing mass vaccination programs, and someone who is directly immersed in the day-to-day operations of the COVID-19 vaccine clinical trials, it my hope that this book will provide a practical basis for individual and family decision making concerning use of COVID-19 vaccines. I will demystify the methods by which the COVID-19 vaccines are being developed and tested, explain the various scientifically based safety strategies being used, and consider the vaccine options available. The final choices are yours and yours alone, but hopefully, this information will help inform these choices with the necessary and appropriate contextual information.

Let us begin our journey.

CHAPTER 1

Vaccine Development

My friends and family all know that I am working on COVID-19 vaccine clinical trials, and so I am always asked: Which vaccine is best? What is the difference between the vaccines? Are the vaccines really safe? I always start my explanation from the beginning, namely, a review of some basics surrounding vaccine development.

Vaccine development can start at a research lab, medical center, small biotechnology company ort a large pharmaceutical company. At any one time, teams of scientists may be working in parallel to develop vaccines against the same pathogen, either a virus or bacteria. Such has been the case with the race to develop a COVID-19 vaccine against the SARS-CoV-2 virus (the virus causing COVID-19), and this undertaking has been carried out at a historic scale in terms of both manpower and resources.

One of the very first steps in the path from lab to clinic is proof-of-concept. A COVID-19 vaccine candidate must prove viable in several early, pre-clinical animal model experiments to verify a potent immune response. This means the body develops the ability for active immunity as a result of the vaccine. Usually, this proof-of-concept evidence involves immunizing mice or other animal models to evaluate a variety of responses (humoral and cellular) appropriate to the vaccine's mechanism of action. Care is taken to document any adverse immune reactions or toxicities.

In some cases, such as with the Pfizer/BioNTech vaccine, additional non-human primate testing, in rhesus macaques, is also done. The study in this case challenged the primates with actual SARS-CoV-2 infection. In this instance, the vaccine prevented lung infection in 100% of the challenged macaques and cleared the nose of detectable virus RNA in 100% of the macaques, as well. With good mouse data, and ideally with additional primate data, a vaccine may be approved by both the governing regulatory body (e.g., the Food and Drug Administration or FDA) and an Institutional Review Board (IRB) to protect the interest of human volunteers, and then be used in a clinical trial.

Clinical trials are usually broken into three distinct phases of escalating size and cost. Phase 1 clinical trials usually involve up to 100 healthy adult volunteers. This type of clinical trial is designed to answer two main questions: does this new vaccine confer the expected immunity and is it safe.

Phase 2 clinical trials may involve several hundred volunteers, where a small proportion of the study group are given placebos, to determine the appropriate dose of vaccine that should be administered. During this trial, the safety of the vaccine is also carefully studied by comparing the control and placebo groups for reactogenicity -- fever, chills, pain or swelling/redness at the injection site, muscle aches, etc. – and other untoward effects.

A Phase 3 clinical trial is the last stage prior to a company being able to request permission from the government regulatory agency (such as the FDA) to be allowed to bring the vaccine into the market and used by designated at-risk individuals. Phase 3 clinical trial are conducted to determine the safety and efficacy of the vaccine. Thousands of participants participate in the Phase 3 study, and this group of volunteers should always be as similar as possible to the population that will be administered the vaccine in real-world situations.

Phase 3 studies are almost always randomized, double-blind, and placebo-controlled, meaning that neither the volunteers nor researchers know who is in the vaccinated or control group. This is critical, as no one working with the volunteers, or the volunteers themselves, should know which ones received the vaccine, lest the results become biased. An example of bias could be if those knowing they received the vaccine had a stronger tendency to report medical problems. Only after the study code is broken can investigators know which subject got the vaccine and which received the placebo. Often, if the vaccine is proven safe and effective and approved by the FDA, arrangements are made to offer the vaccine to those who received the placebo.

The precise number of participants required for a Phase 3 trial is determined though statistical calculation. There needs to be a large enough number of volunteers coming down with COVID-19 during the time of the trial to prove that the vaccine prevents disease when comparing a study population receiving the vaccine, known as the treatment arm, to those receiving a placebo, known as the placebo arm. Another component of a COVID -19 vaccine trial is the clinical site locations, which are ideally set up in areas, or among high-risk popultions, where there are enough new COVID-19 cases naturally circulating in the community to show statistically relevant evidence of vaccine success.

Let's look at how the size of a Phase 3 COVID-19 vaccine is calculated and why they are so large. The number of new cases over a time period per 100,000 population is called the incidence rate of disease. As SARS-CoV-2 virus circulates, and incidence increases, symptomatic and asymptomatic cases can be tested for in the community. This results in a percent positive, or positivity rate, the number of new cases diagnosed with COVID-19 infection divided by the total number tested, multiplied by 100.

We try as best we can to select communities for the trials which have higher than average circulation of virus i.e., a positivity rate of 2% or higher, in order that enough cases of disease are captured during the course of the trial. We also take into account the percentage of the population that has already been infected by COVID-19, with clinical or subclinical disease, resulting in circulating antibodies or a seroprevalence rate, which we estimate to be 10% on average at the present time.

For the study to show a vaccine efficacy of 50% or greater the study population should accrue approximately 150 cases of COVID-19 during the course of the study. Taking all this into account the numbers of volunteers required in an individual COVID-19 vaccine Phase 3 study must be at least 30,000 volunteers, but can range as high as 60,000, if we wish to show that the vaccine is achieving 50% efficacy with 90% confidence, the benchmark set by the FDA for a COVID-19 vaccine to be considered for approval. It is important to note that the clinical studies for COVID-19 vaccines are case driven, meaning that once a sufficient number of community-acquired COVID-19 cases have been reported in study volunteers, the clinical trial may be stopped, and results evaluated by an independent Data Safety Monitoring Board (DSMB) to calculate the vaccine efficacy and assess its safety profile.

To expedite the completion of COVID-19 vaccine trials, hefty development funding and innovative, combined-phase protocols have been used to save valuable development time without any sacrifice in safety. As for funding, in the extraordinary effort to bring a COVID-19 vaccine forward in as short of a time as possible (vaccine clinical trial programs may span five years or longer), decisions have been taken by both vaccine company sponsors and government agencies to spend much larger sums of money on Phase 3 trials in order to have 100 or more vaccine research locations operating in parallel. With this enhanced effort, trial sizes can increase from an average of 10,000 volunteers per study to as many as 60,000! With more sites and more volunteers in these studies, which require capturing enough subjects exposed to COVID-19 to prove effectiveness, clinical trials can be completed more quickly than normal while maintaining safety standards.

Normally, significant time elapses between clinical trial phases and even between subsets within a phase, predominantly because of the needs to pause and analyze the information, present the information to the FDA, have meetings with the FDA, and get approval for the next phase. In the case of the COVID-19 pandemic, the FDA has been working closely with private vaccine manufactures in an extraordinarily collaborative manner to reduce these pauses in activity while not cutting corners on collecting and appropriately analyzing the trial data.

Likewise, in the quest to develop a COVID-19 vaccine as rapidly as possible, Phase 1 and Phase 2 studies are allowed to overlap sequentially into trials called a Phase 1/2 or a Phase 2/3. Although there is a pause after the Phase 1 subset to examine the safety of the vaccine, if deemed safe, the trial can proceed seamlessly into the Phase 2. In other words, rather than stopping the Phase 1 and starting a completely new Phase 2 trial, the study sponsors merely continue the initial study by adding additional participants, thereby saving valuable time.

In these huge Phase 3 trials, participants are carefully monitored to see who develops COVID-19, as determined by both symptoms and laboratory testing for virus. Subjects with symptoms consistent with COVID-19, and having positive test results, are always provided with the best available treatment at independent locations chosen by the subject themselves and outside of the clinical trial. Observation of the subjects is maintained throughout the full length of the trials, which can last two years. This monitoring is essential to determine if the vaccine generated enough immunity to prevent mild, moderate or severe disease, as well as to provide longer-term safety data.

As for safety metrics during the COVID-19 clinical trials, all adverse events are reviewed by a dedicated safety team and reviewed in an unblinded fashion by the study's Data Safety Management Board. For any severe adverse events, a thorough investigation is conducted. Safety endpoints include (a) solicited local and systemic adverse reactions through day 7 (b) unsolicited adverse events through 28 days and (c) medically attended adverse events, adverse events of special interest, and severe adverse events any time within the two-year follow-up.

To assure that vaccines work in the populations most at risk from COVID-19, as well as to bolster confidence that the vaccine will work well when given to the population at large, clinical trials have explicit parameters for enrollment of volunteers with high risk factors for more serious disease (e.g., being over 65 years of age, having specified chronic disease co-morbidities such as diabetes, or being a member of a racial or ethnic minority).

An excellent reference on the basics has been written by Johns Hopkins University's Coronavirus Resource Center, which can be accessed at the link below.
https://coronavirus.jhu.edu/vaccines

To provide transparency and maintain public trust in the COVID-19 vaccine safety, in an unprecedented move, each of the major vaccine companies has released its own clinical trial protocol of their Phase 3 trial to the public. For additional detail, below is a list of these key clinical trial protocols. These documents provide valuable insights into how carefully a clinical trial is planned and all of the safety mechanisms built in.

Pfizer/BioNTech
https://pfe-pfizercom-d8-prod.s3.amazonaws.com/2020-11/C4591001_Clinical_Protocol_Nov2020.pdf

Moderna
https://www.modernatx.com/sites/default/files/mRNA-1273-P301-Protocol.pdf

Novavax
https://www.novavax.com/resources#protocols

AstraZeneca/Oxford
https://s3.amazonaws.com/ctr-med-7111/D8110C00001/52bec400-80f6-4c1b-8791-0483923d0867/c8070a4e-6a9d-46f9-8c32-cece903592b9/D8110C00001_CSP-v2.pdf

Johnson & Johnson / Janssen
https://www.jnj.com/coronavirus/covid-19-phase-3-study-clinical-protocol

CHAPTER 2

The Four Types of Vaccines

I n addition to understanding the nature of clinical trials, I would also like to review how different types of vaccines work, as they each have unique characteristics, which help explain why one approach may work better in some persons than others, or why certain vaccine candidates require more extensive safety review before approval. Some types of COVID-19 candidate vaccines are of a traditional variety, while others are more novel in mechanism. Although there may be slightly different ways to classify vaccines, I have neatly divided them into five basic categories.

Inactivated Virus Vaccines

Inactivation of wild (disease-causing) virus is a staple of vaccine manufacturing and is used for vaccines against diseases such as influenza, hepatitis A, and rabies. The technique of inactivation makes the virus unable to multiply or cause disease. This approach allows the immune system to be exposed to viral proteins and immunity to develop. The antibodies produced by immune cells exposed to the inactivated virus are thereby available to fight off disease when there is later exposure to the active virus.

Making inactivated vaccines requires growing the virus in large quantities first. The virus is then purified and inactivated with chemicals. Inactivated vaccines often require booster doses to improve and sustain immunity. Difficulties in producing a safe and effective vaccine in this manner include the fact that the virus has to be completely inactive, while not changing the virus enough to weaken the immune response. It also must not be inactivated in such a way to create an abnormal and harmful immune response upon exposure to the natural virus.

Inactivated COVID-19 vaccines have been developed outside of the US, e.g., in Russia and China. Such vaccines have already been approved for use in those countries in advance of large Phase 3 studies being published in peer-reviewed medical journals. These countries are immunizing millions of persons while surveilling the populations for adverse events at the same time. With such lax safety standards, these vaccines are not going to be approved for use in the United States.

Live Attenuated Vaccines (LAV)

Live virus vaccines are derived from "wild," or disease-causing, viruses or bacteria. These wild viruses or bacteria are attenuated, or weakened, in a laboratory, usually by repeated culturing. A relatively small dose of virus is administered, creating enough of the organism to stimulate an immune response, and then is rapidly cleared by the immune system.

The immune response to a live attenuated vaccine is virtually identical to that produced by a natural infection. The immune system does not differentiate between an infection from a weakened vaccine virus and an infection from a wild virus. Another positive feature is that the use of an adjuvant (a substance that enhances the body's immune response to an antigen) is usually not required. A small percentage of recipients do not respond to the first dose of an injected live vaccine (such as MMR or varicella), and so a second dose is recommended to provide a very high level of immunity in the population.

Currently available live attenuated viral vaccines include measles, mumps, rubella, varicella, zoster (which contains the same virus as varicella vaccine but in a much higher amount), and influenza (using an intranasal route of delivery). The generation of an attenuated strain of a pathogen for use as a vaccine requires demonstration of its inability to revert genetically to become disease-causing or pathogenic. This is particularly challenging in the case of coronaviruses, as they are known to recombine in nature, and an attenuated vaccine strain could, in theory, recombine with wild coronaviruses to recreate a pathogenic strain. Thus, great care must be taken in design and manufacturing of this type of vaccine.

Live Attenuated Virus COVID-19 vaccines are currently being clinically tested by Meissa, Codagenix and other vaccine compnies. For safety's sake and for example, Meissa vaccines use a molecularly attenuated respiratory syncytial virus (RSV) as the vehicle rather than the SARS-CoV-2 virus.

Protein-Based Vaccines

These kinds of vaccines include viral proteins and no genetic material. Whole proteins or pieces of viral proteins can be used. In COVID-19 vaccines, the key protein of interest is the so-called "spike" protein, which binds to the cells in which the virus replicates at the receptor binding domain. Protein vaccines have a long history of safety and effectiveness in use; for example, vaccines against hepatitis B, shingles and pertussis (whooping cough).

Protein vaccines are often combined with adjuvants to improve the immune response to vaccines. These adjuvants can include aluminum-containing particles, lipids and synthetic forms of DNA, nanoparticles made of cholesterol, phospholipids, and saponins from the soap bark tree – all of which may be used to actually deliver the proteins to cells of the immune system. Adjuvants can be the cause of short-lived local reactions such as redness, swelling and pain at the injection site, as well as fever, chills and body aches. The use of adjuvants in this kind of vaccine is essential for generating a sufficient immune response, including the CD8 T-cell response, to destroy virus-infected cells. New adjuvants are being developed to enhance immune response further and use of any such adjuvant goes through careful clinical trials, as well.

Protein-based COVID-19 vaccines are being clinically tested, for example, by the vaccine companies Novavax and Sanofi.

Viral Vector Vaccines

These vaccines utilize harmless non-replicating or replicating viruses as a vehicle to transfer genetic material, inserting genetic codes for the SARS-CoV-2 spike protein into specific host cells. These host cells can then produce the viral proteins that generate an immune response. The current crop of COVID-19 vaccines includes those using a weakened, non-disease-causing adenovirus or measles virus. Often these viruses do not replicate in the body because specific genes for that replication have been deleted in the laboratory. The first viral vector vaccine was recently approved in 2020 by the European Commission to fight Ebola.

Viral Vector COVID-19 vaccines are being clinically tested by the vaccine companies AstraZeneca (together with Oxford University), Johnson & Johnson / Janssen, and Merck, among others.

Genetic Vaccines: mRNA and DNA

Another approach for vaccine development is to directly deliver the SARS-CoV-2 virus spike protein's genetic blueprint directly into cells as either mRNA (messenger RNA) or DNA. Immediately upon release of the genetic sequence of SARS-CoV-2 to the scientific community, many vaccine scientists turned to existing, albeit novel, vaccine platforms to deliver the genetic material. Up until then, several of these approaches had been used to develop vaccines targeting both infectious diseases and cancer and were in various stages of clinical trials already.

Genetic vaccines do not require cultivation of virus in cells. For mRNA, genetic material can be delivered using lipid nanoparticles to bring mRNA directly into the cells to provide the blueprint for protein creation. For DNA, one uses a DNA plasmid to directly reach into the host cell's nucleus. The assembled protein generates specific immune responses, including the innate immune response (which is perhaps the earliest immune response the body mounts in natural exposure to a pathogen), as well as the more traditionally measured antibody response. No mRNA or DNA vaccine has ever been licensed, although there is considerable human experience using these type vaccines in clinical studies. Pfizer/BioNTech's COVID-19 vaccine was the first mRNA vaccine to receive Emergency Use Authorization.

Genetic COVID-19 vaccines have been developed by the vaccine compnies Moderna, CureVac, Inovio, the Imperial College of London and others.

Additional resources on types of vaccines are listed below.
https://coronavirus.jhu.edu/vaccines
https://www.nature.com/articles/s41577-020-00434-6
https://www.scientificamerican.com/article/genetic-engineering-could-make-a-covid-19-vaccine-in-months-rather-than-years1/
https://www.nejm.org/doi/full/10.1056/nejmoa2022483

CHAPTER 3

Operation Warp Speed

Government oversight is required to combat a global threat such as COVID-19. Operation Warp Speed (OWS) was a Herculean effort bringing together key government agencies with private industry to accelerate response to and control of the COVID-19 pandemic. Among its priorities was advancing development, manufacturing, and distribution of vaccines. As explained by its leaders, Drs. Moncef Slaoui and Mathew Hepburn, in the *New England Journal of Medicine*, OWS provided support to promising vaccine candidates and facilitated the expeditious, parallel execution of the necessary steps toward approval or authorization of safe COVID-19 vaccines by the FDA.

The initiative set ambitious objectives: to deliver tens of millions of doses of a COVID-19 vaccine, with demonstrated safety and efficacy and approved or authorized by the FDA for use in the US population, beginning at the end of 2020, and to have as many as 300 million doses of such vaccines available and deployed by mid-2021. The pace and scope of such a vaccine effort was unprecedented.

The strategy taken was more like that of an investment banker than a government agency: building a diverse project portfolio of vaccines, some of which may fail in testing, that includes at least two vaccine candidates based on each of the four major viable vaccine technologies, or platforms, discussed earlier, for a total of at least eight different vaccines. Given the pandemic situation, such diversification of candidate vaccines reduces the risk of failure due to safety, efficacy, manufacturability or delays, and increases the chance that at least one selected vaccine will succeed.

Additional Information can be found here.
https://www.nejm.org/doi/full/10.1056/NEJMp2027405

CHAPTER 4

*Vaccine Approval: Emergency Use
Authorization vs. Full Licensure*

I n my career, I have had to interact with a wide variety of regulatory agencies. While not usually noted for their speed or innovation, my experience with the FDA has been that in a crisis, they can act expeditiously in close coordination with sister agencies and the expert scientific community. Let's review how the FDA handles new vaccines in the instance of a pandemic.

The US Food and Drug Administration (FDA)

The FDA must approve a vaccine before it can be used in the United States. FDA regulations for the development of vaccines ensure their safety, purity, potency, and effectiveness. FDA also inspects vaccine manufacturing sites to make sure they comply with current Good Manufacturing Practice (cGMP) regulations. Activities related to vaccines are coordinated in its Center for Biologics Evaluation and Research (CBER).

To best advise the FDA, a specialized Vaccines and Related Biological Products Advisory Committee (VBRPAC) makes recommendations to CBER on a vaccine's safety and efficacy prior to approval. In all cases to-date, its recommendations are followed by the Commissioner of the FDA, who has the final legal authority to release a vaccine into use. The Committee consists of 15 voting members selected from among authorities knowledgeable in the fields of immunology, molecular biology, virology, vaccine development, preventive medicine, infectious diseases, and pediatrics. The committee meets in open, publicly broadcast meetings where anyone can hear the experts discuss the data.

There are two different paths by which a vaccine can enter the market in order to address the COVID-19 pandemic. The first pathway is by use of a so-called "Emergency Use Authorization" (EUA) from the FDA, based on data submitted to the FDA by the vaccine manufacturer. The second is by full licensure of the vaccine by the FDA in response to a complete Biologics Licensure Application (BLA) from the vaccine manufacturer.

Reviewing the FDA's own published guidance documents, a COVID-19 vaccine perfectly fits the EUA scenario envisioned for this alternative and usually temporary status. To obtain emergency use authorization for marketing a COVID-19 vaccine, four criteria must be satisfied:

• First, the disease agent, in this case SARS-CoV-2, must cause a serious or life-threatening disease. The COVID-19 pandemic certainly does.

• Secondly, it should be reasonable to believe that the vaccine may be effective to prevent COVID-19, based on the totality of scientific evidence available, including data from adequate and well controlled trials. This is precisely the data that is being obtained through properly designed Phase 3 clinical trials.

• Thirdly, the known and potential benefits of the vaccine must outweigh the known and potential risks. This safety data is also coming from a series of well-designed clinical trials.

• Lastly, there is no adequate, approved, and available alternative vaccine for preventing COVID-19. At this point, there are no fully licensed COVID-19 vaccines.

Thus, as of now, all four elements needed for EUA consideration are satisfied. In the case of investigational vaccines being developed for the prevention of COVID-19, any assessment regarding an EUA is made on a case-by-case basis considering the target population, the characteristics of the vaccine, the pre-clinical and human clinical study data on the vaccine, and the totality of the available scientific evidence relevant to the vaccine.

As explained by vaccine experts Drs Philip Krause and Marion Gruber in the *New England Journal of Medicine*, COVID-19 vaccines approved under the EUA guidance should have significant benefits as well as sufficient data to assess the safety profile. They rightly point out that the public's entire confidence in a vaccine depends on the quality of the clinical science used to evaluate it.

It is not in public or private interest to immediately rush a vaccine candidate to approval after clinical trial success in meeting the disease prevention endpoint without assuring its safety from a holistic standpoint. Such steps include a two-month median follow-up after completion of the full vaccination regimen. This allows identification of potential adverse events that were not apparent in the immediate post-vaccination period during the Phase 3 clinical trial, and will also provide greater confidence in their absence, if none are observed. EUA authorization is conditional upon continued monitoring of vaccine safety in those vaccinated as they complete the entire monitoring period specified in the trial protocol, often two years.

Following the EUA approval process, full licensure would be the next step. The FDA generally requires at least six months of safety follow-up for serious and other medically significant adverse events in a sufficient number of vaccinees. Given the immediate need for high-risk groups to have an effective vaccine, vaccine companies take the EUA route once their successful Phase 3 data becomes available.

Below is an article with additional information on the approval process.
https://www.nejm.org/doi/full/10.1056/NEJMp2031373

CHAPTER 5

Vaccine Safety Monitoring: Post-Authorization or Licensure

Wearing my public health hat, I support the prevailing opinion that nothing can be more critical than reviewing the ongoing safety of vaccines once they have been released to the public through either the EUA or full licensure pathways. This is accomplished through multiple governmental programs, admittedly a jumble of names and acronyms. Luckily for us, many of these initiatives are mutually reinforcing and provide a national safety net to uncover and address any issues that arise.

Dr Grace Lee at Stanford University and her colleagues have highlighted many of these safety mechanisms in the *Journal of the American Medical Association (JAMA)*, as described below.
https://jamanetwork.com/journals/jama/fullarticle/2772137

Other aspects of the national vaccine safety program have been detailed at the emergency VBRPAC meeting held by the FDA concerning the COVID-19 Vaccine.
https://www.fda.gov/advisory-committees/advisory-committee-calendar/vaccines-and-related-biological-products-advisory-committee-october-22-2020-meeting-announcement#event-materials

The Centers for Disease Control and Prevention (CDC)
The CDC is the national public health institute in the United States under the Department of Health and Human Services. The CDC's overall responsibility is to address health, safety, and se-

curity threats of Americans both at home and abroad. The CDC is focused on vaccine planning, working closely with health departments and partners to prepare for when a vaccine is available.

The Advisory Committee on Immunization Practices (ACIP)
The ACIP develops recommendations on how to use vaccines under the auspices of the CDC. These recommendations are then passed to the Director of the CDC. The panel itself is composed of independent vaccine experts, most of who come from the academic milieu, and is staffed by CDC epidemiologists. There are many non-voting liaison members representing major medical professional associations and government agencies. For example, liaisons represent the American Academy of Pediatrics and the American College of Physicians.

A newly constituted COVID-19 Vaccine Safety Technical (VaST) Working Group advises the ACIP COVID-19 Vaccine Workgroup and the full ACIP on the safety of COVID-19 vaccines in development and post-approval. This panel is composed of experts in coronavirus, clinical trials and vaccine safety, and representatives of various agencies with experience in vaccine safety, such as the FDA, the Veterans Administration and the CDC. Very importantly, the ACIP develops the CDC's recommended prioritization system for distribution of COVID-19 vaccines.

The Vaccine Adverse Event Reporting System (VAERS)
VAERS is a surveillance system that relies on reporting by patients or family members, healthcare professionals, or manufacturers to rapidly detect temporally associated, potential adverse events after vaccination. A national system, its scope includes all 320 million US residents as its covered population, i.e., all ages, races, jurisdictions, health statuses, etc. VAERS staff review individual case reports, but the organization also utilizes statistical data mining methods to detect disproportionate reporting of specific vaccine-adverse event combinations. A commitment has been made to minimize any delay in analysis and to provide the CDC and FDA with daily updates.

The Vaccine Safety Datalink (VSD)
VSD is a 30-year collaboration between the CDC and nine national health systems that uses healthcare encounter data and electronic medical records to capture data on vaccines and potential outcomes of interest in a well-defined population of approximately 11.3 million insured patients, with near real-time capabilities for signal detection.

v-Safe
v-Safe is a new smartphone-based active surveillance program developed for the COVID-19 vaccine. It uses text messaging to initiate web-based survey monitoring. conducts electronic health checks on vaccine recipients daily for the first week post-vaccination, and then weekly thereafter until six weeks post-vaccination. Active telephone follow-up is completed through the VAERS program for people reporting clinically important events during any v-safe health check.

CHAPTER 6

Authorized and Other Leading
COVID-19 Vaccines

At the heart of this booklet is an attempt to familiarize the potential vaccine recipient about the vaccines they might receive, their safety and their effectiveness. We are fortunate that a variety of COVID-19 vaccines have been authorized under EUA, or in advanced clinical trials with EUAs on the horizon. These vaccines are not interchangeable, because each one works differently; however, none is being released without solid scientific and clinical evidence. Let's review each of the major vaccines in detail, giving you the best available data on which to make personal decisions.

Pfizer and BioNTech (mRNA Vaccine)

Pfizer, the New York-based global pharmaceutical behemoth, and BioNTech, a smaller biotechnology company based in Germany, teamed up early in the pandemic to produce a COVID-19 vaccine. This mRNA vaccine, called BNT16b2, was the very first vaccine to have its results submitted to the FDA for EUA authorization setting off a frenzied effort to prepare for immunizing millions of people across the US and around the world. On December 11, 2020 the FDA announced this vaccine was the first one authorized for use under an EUA, based on the recommendation of the Vaccine and Related Biologics Products Advisory Committee of experts held the day prior. This vaccine candidate was found, in the FDA's own review of the Pfizer/BioNTech Phase 3 clinical trial data to be 95.0% effective in preventing COVID-19 in persons 16 years of age and older.

Safety data from approximately 38,000 participants ≥16 years of age, randomized 1:1 to vaccine or placebo with a median of 2 months of follow up after the second dose, suggested a favorable safety profile, with no specific safety concerns identified that would preclude issuance of an EUA. Available safety data from all participants enrolled through the November 14, 2020 data cut-off point (with 43,252 volunteers and which includes late enrollment of additional adolescent and adult participants), was consistent with the safety profile for the approximately 38,000 participants with median follow-up of 2 months and also did not raise specific safety concerns. The most common solicited adverse reactions were minor injection site reactions (84.1%), fatigue (62.9%), headache (55.1%), muscle pain (38.3%), chills (31.9%), joint pain (23.6%), fever (14.2%); severe adverse reactions occurred in 0.0% to 4.6% of participants, were more frequent after Dose 2 than after Dose 1, and were generally less frequent in participants ≥55 years of age (≤ 2.8%) as compared to younger participants (≤4.6%).

Approximately 42% of global participants and 30% of US participants came from racially and ethnically diverse backgrounds, and 41% of global and 45% of US participants were 56-85 years of age. The trial will continue to collect efficacy and safety data in participants for an additional two years.

The companies have developed specially designed, temperature-controlled thermal shippers utilizing dry ice to maintain temperature conditions of -70°C±10°C. They can be used be as temporary storage units for 15 days by refilling with dry ice. Each shipper contains a GPS-enabled thermal sensor to track the location and temperature of each vaccine shipment across pre-set routes leveraging Pfizer's broad distribution network.
https://www.fda.gov/media/144245/download

Moderna Therapeutics (mRNA Vaccine)

Moderna, a biotechnology company in Massachusetts, became the second vaccine given an EUA authorization by the FDA. Several years prior to the pandemic, Moderna had previously put forward an mRNA vaccine technology platform that could provide advantages in efficacy, speed of development, and production scalability and reliability. This preparation enabled rapid deployment of the platform for their COVID-19 vaccine, co-developed with investigators from the National Institutes for Allergy and Infectious Diseases' Vaccine Research Center, an arm of the National Institutes of Health.

Prior to its EUA, Moderna announced that the independent, NIH-appointed Data Safety Monitoring Board (DSMB) for the Phase 3 study of mRNA-1273, its vaccine candidate against COVID-19, informed Moderna that the trial met the statistical criteria pre-specified in the study protocol for efficacy, with a vaccine efficacy of 94.5%.

The primary endpoint of the Phase 3 study was based on the analysis of COVID-19 cases confirmed and adjudicated starting two weeks following the second dose of vaccine. This first interim analysis was based on 95 cases, of which 90 cases of COVID-19 were observed in the placebo group versus 5 cases observed in the mRNA-1273 group, resulting in a point estimate of vaccine efficacy of 94.5% (p <0.0001).

A secondary endpoint analyzed severe cases of COVID-19 and included 11 severe cases in this first interim analysis. All 11 cases occurred in the placebo group and none in the mRNA-1273 vaccinated group. The 95 COVID-19 cases included 15 older adults (ages 65+) and 20 participants identifying as being from diverse communities (including 12 Hispanic or Latinx, 4 Black or African Americans, 3 Asian Americans and 1 multiracial).

The interim analysis included a concurrent review of the available Phase 3 study safety data by the DSMB, which did not report any significant safety concerns. A review of solicited adverse events indicated that the vaccine was generally well tolerated. The majority of adverse events were mild or moderate in severity. Side effects events greater than or equal to 2% in frequency after the first dose included injection site pain (2.7%), and after the second dose included fatigue (9.7%), muscle aches (8.9%), joint pain (5.2%), headache (4.5%), pain (4.1%) and erythema/redness at the injection site (2.0%). These solicited adverse events were generally short-lived. Moderna has announced its expectation to be able to produce 500 million-1 billion doses worldwide in 2021.

https://investors.modernatx.com/news-releases/news-release-details/modernas-covid-19-vaccine-candidate-meets-its-primary-efficacy

Johnson & Johnson (Viral Vector Vaccine)

The Johnson & Johnson (J&J) vaccine candidate known as JNJ-78436735 or Ad26.COV2.S is a recombinant viral vector vaccine that uses a human adenovirus to express the SARS-CoV-2 spike protein in cells. While adenoviruses are a group of viruses that cause the common cold, the adenovirus vector used in the vaccine candidate has been modified so that it can no longer replicate in humans and cause disease. J&J uses the same vector in the first dose of its prime-boost vaccine regimen against Ebola virus disease (Ad26.ZEBOV and MVA-BN-Filo), which was previously granted marketing authorization by the European Commission.

Unlike the Pfizer/BioNTech and Moderna vaccines, which store genetic information in single stranded RNA, the Johnson & Johnsone vaccine uses double-stranded DNA. Adenovirus-based vaccines are more hearty than mRNA vaccines. DNA is not as fragile as mRNA. Adenovirus's tough protein coat helps protect the genetic material. As a result, the Johnson & Johnson vaccine can be refrigerated for up to three months at 36-46 °F (2-8 ° C).

Unlike other vaccine candidates, the J&J vaccine is a 1-dose regimen, greatly simplifying the vaccine schedule. Results from the Phase 1/2 trial, published in the New England Journal of Medicine, showed the vaccine induced neutralizing antibodies (the most potent kind) in over 90% of volunteers at day 29 and in over 100% of volunteers aged 18-55 at day 57. Those antibodies remained stable through day 71, the latest time point measured in this study. For volunteers over 65 years, antibodies were induced in 96% by day 29, the last day they were follwed in this group at time of publication.

In terms of safety, this study demonstrated injection site (local) and systemic reactions to vaccinations either occured on the day of vaccination or the next day, and generally resolved within 24 hours. The most common adverse events (mild-to-moderate) were fatigue, headache, muscle pain and injection site pain. Side effects like these were lower in the older age group. One participant visited a hospital for fever associated with the vaccination but recovered within 12 hours.

Based on these extraordinary early results from a one-dose vaccine, Johnson & Johnson completed enrollment of a 45,000-person Phase 3 study across the US, Brazil, Argentina, Chile, Columbia, Mexico, Peru and South Africa. Results have been submitted for EUA but not yet publicly available. A second Phase 3 study is being launched to see if a 2-dose regimen might increase the durability of protection.

https://www.nejm.org/doi/full/10.1056/NEJMoa2034201

AstraZeneca / University of Oxford (Viral Vector Vaccine)

AstraZeneca, a global pharmaceutical company based in Cambridge, England, has developed a COVID-19 vaccine called AZD1222. The vaccine was co-invented by the University of

Oxford and its spinoff company, Vaccitech. It uses a chimpanzee specific virus vector based on a weakened version of a common cold virus (adenovirus) which cannot replicate. After vaccination, a SARS-CoV-2 virus surface spike protein is produced, priming the immune system to attack the SARS-CoV-2 virus if it later infects the body.

AstraZeneca and Oxford University have released interim results from their Phase 3 study conducted in the UK and Brazil. It showed that when the vaccine was given in a one-half dose followed by a full booster dose regimen (in 2,741 subjects), vaccine efficacy was 90%. When another schedule was used, a full dose followed by a full booster dose (in 895 subjects), efficacy dropped to 62%, for an average efficacy of 70%. An Independent Data Safety Monitoring Board determined the analysis met the study's primary endpoint showing protection from COVID-19 occurring 14 days or more after the second dose. No serious safety events related to the vaccine have been confirmed. Emergency Use Authorization is being submitted to the World Health Organization, while the results of additional Phase 3 trials totaling 60,000 subjects globally, including the US, are still pending.
https://www.astrazeneca.com/media-centre/press-releases/2020/azd1222hlr.html

CHAPTER 7

Other Major COVID-19 Candidate
Vaccines in Development

Hopefully, a number of additional vaccines will be able to complete the full range of clinical trials. This will not only provide a greater global supply, but it may turn out that some of these vaccines are particularly effective in protecting specific high-risk populations such as the elderly, who often have a harder time mounting protective immune response to traditional vaccines. Below, I provide some information on a few of the other vaccines already in clinical trials.

CureVac (mRNA Vaccine)
CureVac's vaccine includes mRNA coding for a stabilized form of the spike protein and contains it in a lipid nanoparticle. CureVac announced that their Phase 1 data, using a two-dose regimen, demonstrated no serious vaccine-related adverse events. The immune response was comparable to that seen in persons who have recently recovered from COVID-19 disease. As a result, the company decided to move forward with their Phase 2/3 clinical trial. CureVac has negotiated a deal to provide the European Union with up to 250 million doses of their vaccine. They project manufacturing up to 300 million doses and up to 600 million doses the following year.

Arcturus / Duke NUS (mRNA Vaccine)
The California-based company Arcturus and Duke-NUS Medical School in Singapore have developed an mRNA vaccine having

a "self-replicating" design that leads to a greater production of viral proteins. Tests on animals showed that it protected them against infection. In August, Arcturus launced a Phase 1/2 trial at Singapore General Hospital. The company subsequently announced that an interim analysis of the trial showed that the vaccine produced an immune response that was in the range of responses seen in people who recovered from COVID-19. Singapore has reached an agreement with Arcturus to spend up to $175 million to acquire vaccines.

Inovio (DNA Vaccine)

The Inovio DNA-based vaccine is delivered into the skin with electrical pulses from a hand-held device that allows the DNA itself to enter specific cells. Inovio announced interim data from a Phase 1 study in which they found no serious adverse effects and measured a satisfactory immune response in 34 out of 36 volunteers. Subsequently, Inovio was given the green light by the FDA to proceed with their 40-subject Phase 2 as part of their Phase 2/3 trial plan. The vaccine uses a two-dose regimen and does not require a frozen cold chain for transportation and storage.

Merck (Viral Vector Vaccine)

Merck's vaccine uses a modified measles virus to deliver antigens to the immune system. The vaccine, V591, was obtained via the acquisition of Themis, a biotechnology company, which licenses the viral vaccine from the famed Institut Pasteur in France. The vaccine is being tested in a Phase 1/2 clinical trial of 260 persons in Belgium using both a single and 2-dose regimen.

Merck also is developing a second COVID-19 vaccine in collaboration with IAVI, a global not-for-profit vaccine development group. This vaccine uses a recombinant vesicular stomatitis virus (rVSV) as a vector, the same virus technology Merck used to develop its Ebola Zaire virus vaccine, ERVEBO, which came to market in 2019.

Novavax (Protein Vaccine)

Novavax's vaccine candidate NVX-CoV2373 is a stable protein vaccine delivered using a proprietary nanoparticle technology. Its Phase 3 clinical trial in the UK was composed of 15,000 volunteers and completed enrollment in November 2020, with results expected in 2021. In the Phase 1 portion of its Phase 1/2 in the UK , the vaccine was generally well tolerated, and elicited robust antibody responses numerically superior to those seen in the bloodstream of persons having recently recovered from COVID-19 infection. A second pivotal Phase 3 program is being established for the US and Mexico.

Sanofi (Viral Vector Vaccine)
On September 3, 2020, Sanofi announced a Phase 1/2 clinical trial of its candidate COVID-19 vaccine. The vaccine employs the same recombinant protein-based technology used in their seasonal influenza vaccine, and uses an adjuvant from the company GSK to enhance the immune response. Results from the 440-person Phase 1/2 clinical trial showed the vaccine triggered immune responses in persons aged 18-49 that were comparable to those seen in convelescent plasma. However a low immune response was seen in older adults. An insufficient concentration of the protein antigen was identified as a most likely cause. As a result, new re-formulated version of the vaccine is entering a phase 2 study slated to begin in February 2021.

CHAPTER 8

Distribution of the Vaccine

One of the most contentious and immediately relevant issues is who can get the vaccine and when. After a vaccine is authorized for use, its supply is usually limited due to finite manufacturing capacity, the speed of manufacturing technologies, and the logistical challenges of distribution and administration. During the time between when the vaccine is authorized and when it becomes widely available, planning is required to determine which groups should be prioritized to receive the vaccine first, and which groups can wait until more vaccine doses are produced.

Actual distribution of an approved vaccine is usually the exclusive purview of the vaccine manufacturer, but in the case of the COVID-19 vaccine, the US government has procured millions of doses of vaccine in advance from multiple manufacturers for public distribution. Numerous medical and public health organizations have proposed methods for equitable distribution of this vaccine. The CDC issued its national recommendations for states, as each state individually will be managing the distribution of vaccines provided through the federal government. The CDC's interim COVID-19 Vaccination Playbook for distribution at the State level clearly indicates states should plan for three phases of vaccine distribution: (1) limited COVID-19 vaccine doses available; (2) large number of doses available, supply likely to meet demand; and (3) likely sufficient supply.

https://www.cdc.gov/vaccines/imz-managers/downloads/COVID-19-Vaccination-Program-Interim_Playbook.pdf

Various expert groups have proposed their own distribution plans, including the National Academies of Science, Engineering and Medicine (NAS); the World Health Organization (WHO) Strategic Advisory Groups of Experts (SAGE); and the Advisory Committee on Immunization Practices (ACIP), the federal advisory committee composed of medical and public health experts who develop recommendations on the use of vaccines for the US public.

The proposal I like best, and the one I hope will be consulted by the states, is from the Johns Hopkins Center for Health Security, drafted by a multidisciplinary committee of experts in public health. The framework places emphasis on supporting the common good by promoting public health and by enabling social and economic activity. It also emphasizes the importance of treating individuals fairly while promoting social equity by, for example, addressing racial and ethnic disparities in COVID-19 mortality, and by recognizing the contributions of essential workers who have been overlooked in previous allocation schemes.

The Hopkins proposal recommends priority distribution according to two tiers.

https://www.centerforhealthsecurity.org/our-work/pubs_archive/pubs-pdfs/2020/200819-vaccine-allocation.pdf

Tier 1:
- Those most essential in sustaining the ongoing COVID-19 response
- Those at greatest risk of severe illness and death, and their caregivers
- Those most essential to maintaining core societal functions

Tier 2:
- Those involved in broader health provision

- Those who face greater barriers to access care if they become seriously ill
- Those contributing to maintenance of core societal functions
- Those whose living or working conditions give them elevated risk of infection, even if they have lesser or unknown risk of severe illness and death.

Let's dive deeper into the tiers to determine if you, based on your occupation or health history, might qualify under this tiered system.

Tier 1

- Frontline health workers providing care for COVD-19 patients

- Frontline emergency medical services personnel

- Pandemic vaccine manufacturing and supply chain personnel

- COVID-19 diagnostic and immunization teams

- Public health workers carrying out critical, frontline interventions in the community

- Frontline long-term care providers

- Healthcare workers providing direct care to patients with high-risk conditions

- Adults aged 65 and older and those living with them or otherwise providing care to them

- Individuals with health conditions that put them at significant increased risk of severe COVID-19. According to the CDC, these conditions include: cancer, chronic kidney disease, chronic obstructive pulmonary disease, heart conditions, immunocomprimised states, obesity, pregnancy (as appropriate), sickle cell disease, and type 2 diabetes.

- Members of social groups experiencing high fatality rates

- Other groups yet to be identified who are shown to be at significant risk of severe illness and death

- Frontline public transportation workers

- Teachers and school workers (pre-kindergarten through 12th grade)

Tier 2

- Health workers and staff with direct patient contact (non-COVID-19 specific)

- Pharmacy staff

- Those living in remote locations with substandard infrastructure and health access (Native American reservations, isolated rural communities)

- Frontline workers involved in maintaining operations of electricity, water, sanitation, information, financial, fuel infrastructure (who cannot work remotely)

- Warehouse, delivery workers (including postal workers)

- Deployed military (including National Guard) involved in operations

- Police and fire personnel with frequent public contact

- Transportation Security Administration and border security personnel with direct public contact

- Those unable to maintain safe physical distance within their living or work environments

- Other groups yet to be identified who are shown to be at elevated risk of infection because of other working conditions

With these broad recommendations in mind, it is my strong view that healthcare workers with direct clinical exposure to

COVID-19 patients and those at highest individual medical risk from COVID-19 be at the front of the line. The CDC guidelines, place persons over 75 years of age in Tier 1. Unfortunately some states, perhaps as a result of political pressures, have categorized an overly broad swath of social and occupational groups, even at times medical marijana dispensary employees, as "essential workers" to move them up to the front of the line. Corporations such as Amazon, Lyft, DoorDash and lobyists from specific industries such as airlines, retail, exterminators, are vying for special access to the vaccine.

I hope in practice that those at highest individual medical risk by virture of residence in a nursing home, direct regular frontline interaction with COVID-19 patients, advanced age, or medical conditions which put them at very high personal risk for severe COVID-19, receive limited vaccine first. Inclusion of broader social or occupational groups, which necessarily include many healthy individuals not of high risk for severe disease or death, is for second order discussion and perhaps local prioritization. To me, the guiding principle is to provide vaccination first to the most medically vulnerable persons and utimately save the most lives.

CHAPTER 9

Frequently Asked Questions (FAQs)
about COVID-19 vaccine

I f there is one thing I know from the practice of medicine, it's that answering patients' questions is essential to good communication and trust. Below I have listed a few of the most common quesions about the COVID-19 vaccine and my responses.

Q. Will the vaccine end the pandemic?

A. It has been estimated that immunity of 70% of the country might be required in order to effectively stop widespread ongoing virus transmission. Given the estimated background exposure leading to natural protection of up to 10-20% of the population, this means that an additional 50-60% of the country must still be vaccinated to reach this level. This may not happen until mid-2021, when an adequate vaccine supply can be widely distributed to the general public. However, that is not to say that use of vaccines even at lower overall rates won't play a significant role in protecting large parts of the medically high-risk community. Meanwhile, handwashing, masking and social distancing will continue to play important preventive roles in the foreseeable future.

Q. Usually, vaccines take many years to be developed and tested.

How have several vaccines been able to have been authorized for use in only 10 months?

A. The pandemic has motivated the scientific community as never before. Operation Warp Speed invested billions of dollars into vaccine development and supply. This included the subsidized, parallel manufacturing of different vaccines to expedite completion of clinical trials as well as advance procurement contracts, without sacrificing any of the strict standards around safety in clinical studies or in manufacturing processes. Whereas typical vaccine clinical trials may have tens of sites, with increased resources from the government and the private vaccine companies themselves, hundreds of sites are being utilized simultaneously. Many tens of thousands of volunteers are being immunized in a brief period of time, often over a one-month or six-week period, shortening the time it takes for a clinical study to be completed.

Q. How effective is the vaccine?

A. Currently authorized vaccines have been shown to have approximately 95% effectiveness in preventing COVID-19, and virtually 100% effectiveness in preventing serious outcomes from COVID-19 such as hospitalization and death.

Q. How safe is the vaccine? Are there side effects?

A. The currently authorized vaccines have been shown to be very safe with by and large only transient mild or moderate side effects (redness/sweeling, pain at the injection site, muscle aches, headaches, etc), as detailed earlier in this book, and which pale in comparison with symptomatic COVID-19 itself. A small number of more serious allergic reactions have been reported out of millions of vaccinations, primarily in those with a history of severe allergic reactions, and persons with that medical history should avoid the vaccines until more in known. Moreover, all health providers administering vaccines are required to have emergency plans in place in case of adverse events.

Careful surveillance for less common side effects is taking place as both more people become vaccinated and as the time since vaccination increases. Ongoing monitoring is done by the vaccine companies in their FDA clinical trials for the first two years, while a wide range of well-established health agencies monitor side effects from the moment of initial rollout of vaccinations going forward.

Q. Will there be enough vaccine for everyone?

A. Initially vaccines will be in limited supply. For that reason, states have developed plans to prioritize the vaccines for highest-risk individuals (such as front-line healthcare workers routinely exposed to COVID-19) and those living in the highest-risk situations (such as long-term care facilities for the elderly). As supply gradually increases, the prioritized groups will expand until there is sufficient vaccine availability for persons with high-risk medical conditions, age over 65, and subsequntly the general population. The US government is providing massive sums of money to support scale-up of vaccine manufacturing capability to allow for enough vaccine to cover the entire US population by 2021.

Q. How many shots of COVID-19 vaccine will be needed?

A. All but one of the vaccines that have been authorized and/or are currently in Phase 3 clinical trials require two doses. Other vaccines in development may require only one dose. Whether a booster dose is required remains to be seen, and will be based on long-term data that can tell us the amount of antibody remaining in circulation after various periods of time post-vaccination. If antibodies decline, a booster dose may be required.

Q. How long will the immunity from the vaccine last?

A. It is not known how long antibodies (humoral immunity) will be able to be detected in the blood following the basic dose regimen for each vaccine. However, finding out is one key objective in all Phase 3 clinical trials. These trials will check antibody levels over the two years post-emergency use authorization to determine if and when a booster dose might be advisable. In some cases, thanks to cellular immunity, many of the vaccines may continue to provide partial protection despite low levels of circulating antibodies.

Q. Can I be sure a vaccine is safe is safe when development seems to have been rushed?

A. While the search for vaccines has been the highest priority for scientists and is occurring at a dizzying pace, this does not mean corners have been cut. In all clinical trials, patient safety has been the number one concern. The rapid speed of development can be attributed to several clever design modifications for the trials themselves.

Often, the size of the clinical trials includes about 10,000 volunteers in Phase 3. In the search for COVID-19 vaccines, however, the biostatisticians designing studies have been able to overlap study stop/start dates and increase the size of trials significantly, to 30,000-60,000 volunteers each over a 4-6 week timeline, allowing studies to start earlier and take less time to complete without sacrificing any safety. Also, vaccine scientists don't usually start Phase 2 testing until Phase 1 studies have finished, and similarly don't start Phase 3 until Phase 2 is complete. In the case of COVID-19 vaccines, because of study efficiencies, some overlap of study start days has been possible, with FDA approvals, saving time.

Q. Should I expect side effects from vaccination?

A. The new vaccines, such as from Pfizer/BioNTech and Moderna are extraordinarily safe. Safety data were extensively and independently reviewed by the FDA prior to its recommendation for Emergency Use Authorization. There were some short-lived side effects that might be expected from a highly effective vaccine that is supercharging the immune system, but which a recipient must be prepared for none the less. This includes some redness and /or pain at the injections site (84%), fatigue (63%), headache (55%0, muscle pain (38%), chills (40%), joint pain (23%) and fever (14%). Such side effects were seen less frequently in those at or over 55 years of age. A similar profile is seen with the other mRNA vaccines. These side effects pale in comparison with potential consequences of mild-severe COVID-19. Allergy questions are covered below.

Q. I have occasional mild seasonal allergies. Can I safely use the COVID-19 vaccines?

A. For persons with occasional mild allergies, there is no specific contraindication for vaccination. There have been several cases of severe allergic reactions to the Pfizer/BioNTech COVID-19 vaccine in persons with prior histories of severe allergic reactions (two cases out of 138,000 doses initially distributed in the United Kingdom). In the US, two additional allegeric reactions have been seen in people without that prior medical history, both unusally clustered in Alaska, without apparent explanation although investigations continue.

Allergy experts in the US advise at present that only the rare patient with allergy to specific components of the vaccine, specifically a compound called polyethylene glycol or PEG, shouldn't receive the vaccine. This compound is generally speaking inert and found in ultrasound gels, and laxatives among other commonly used products. Other ingredients, none of which are common allergens, include a mix of salts, fatty substances and sugars that help stabilize the vaccine. Having allegies to foods or oral medications doesn't increase your chance of an allergic reaction to the vaccine.

As a result of these atypical incidents, a clear requirement has been issued that all providers of COVID-19 vaccine have appropriate emergency response capabilities on hand to handle serious allergic reactions and that vaccinees be observed for 15 minutes following vaccination.

Q. Can you still get infected, and infect others, if you got vaccinated?

A. We don't know. Most studies are intended to focus on protecting people from developing symptoms of COVID-19. So, it's not certain that that the vaccine would stop infection or limit spreading the virus to others. This also implies that until we obtain more data from those who are vaccinated we should continue to wear a mask and socially distance.

Q. Can the vaccine give me COVID-19?

A. No. The approved vaccines do not use a whole virus but just snippets of genetic material to spur production of proteins to help trigger the immune system. There is no live SARS-CoV-2 virus in the vaccine to replicate and infect anyone.

Q. How many doses of COVID-19 vaccine will I need?

A. All but one of the COVID-19 vaccines currently in Phase 3 clinical trials in the United States need two shots to be effective. The other COVID-19 vaccine in advanced development, from Johnson & Johnson, uses one shot. Nonetheless, they too are studying the added value of a two dose series to further boost durability of response.

Q. How does the COVID-19 vaccine compare with other vaccines in terms of effectiveness?

A. While COVID-19 vaccines are approximately 95% effective in clinical studies, the flu vaccine, on the other hand, may only have efficacy of 40-60% in any one flu season. Moreover, flu vaccines typically work less well in patients over 65 years of age or in immunocompromised individuals. Despite this, in the 2018-2019 flu season vaccines prevented 4.4 million influenza illnesses, 58,000 influenza-associated hospitalizations, and 3,500 influenza-associated deaths. Thus, we see how important immunization can be. We know the new COVID-19 vaccines work well in older people although studies in immunocompromised individuals have yet to be conducted.

Q. Which vaccine should I take?

A. The new vaccines have not been shown to be interchangeable and each works through a different mechanism, however all the vaccines authorized to-date have high efficacy at approximately 95%. If a two-dose vaccine, it is important to take both doses of the same vaccine, as the first dose may only confer 50% immunity. The vaccine record you will be given will detail which vaccine you took first. Usually returning to the same provider will assure that the same vaccine will be available for your second dose.

Q. What about children and adolescents?

A. The Pfizer vaccine has already been tested in adolescents down to age 16 and thus the emergency use authorization includes this age group. The Moderna vaccine was only tested in persons over 18 years of age and is not being offered to adolescents until such studies can be completed. Other vaccines will have age-appropriate labeling based on the clinical trials data appropriate to the safety data they collect. Efforts are underway to test efficacy and safety of the new vaccines on children 12 years of age and older. After that, testing on children even younger will no doubt be started.

Q. Should I be vaccinated if I have had COVID-19 already?

A. Yes. It's safe, and perhaps even beneficial, for anyone who has had COVID-19 to get the vaccine at some point. Although people who have contracted the virus do have immunity, it is too soon to know how long it lasts. Therefore, it makes sense to get the shot regardless.

Q. Is the vaccine effective in Persons of Color?

A. Yes. Great care is being taken to assure that communities of color are included fully and equitably in all Phase 3 studies of efficacy and safety. For example, in an analysis of data from their vaccine studies, Moderna showed a 97.5% efficacy in persons from communities of color. In that Phase 3 study 10.3% of volunteers identified as Black or African-America, 4.3% were of Asian descent, 0.7% were American Indian or Alaska Native while 20.6% were Hispanic or Latino.

Q. Will the vaccine work in older people?

A. Yes. The Moderna vaccine, in particular, has shown that in those over 65 years of age the vaccine efficacy is 86.4%. The Pfizer vaccine has shown good efficacy as well, but their data is more limited at present. The jury is out for non-mRNA type vaccines which may require special adjuvants (immune enhancing ingredients in the vaccine itself).

CONCLUSIONS

It is sincerely hoped that after reviewing this information you have acquired a better understanding about the careful ways that vaccines are manufactured, tested and evaluated, and you will have confidence that COVID-19 vaccines authorized by the FDA are safe and effective for those most at risk of severe disease progression as well as the general public. Whether authorized via EUA or approved through the full licensure pathway there is a powerful deliberative review process by recognized experts outside of the FDA itself.

The relatively rapid testing of vaccines for COVID-19 is a consequence of specially designed clinical trials that have large numbers of sites and volunteers, and in which study phases overlap without cutting any corners in safety prior to release. I have also tried to answer the most frequently asked questions related to individual decision-making on vaccine use for oneself and one's own family. Let's hope with rapid manufacturing, effective distribution and public acceptance of the vaccines, we can change the course of the pandemic -- saving lives, reducing disease complications and sparing our world from more harmful economic disruption.

ABOUT THE AUTHOR

Zeil Rosenberg M. D.

Zeil Rosenberg M.D. is a Board-Certified Preventive Medicine specialist and physician executive who has devoted much of his life's work to the development and delivery of safe and effective vaccines. Currently, Dr. Rosenberg is directly immersed in the design, patient recruitment and execution of COVID-19 vaccine clinical trials as Medical Director with a global medical research company.

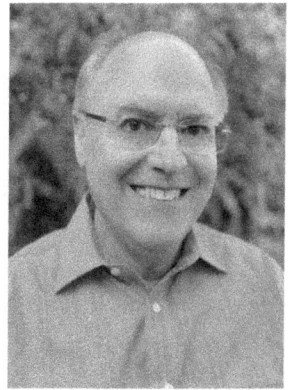

While a Child Survival Fellow at Johns Hopkins University, Dr. Rosenberg served for four years as USAID's Resident Advisor for Immunization at the Indonesian Ministry of Health, where he led efforts to eliminate neonatal tetanus though immunization coverage for all children. Moving to New York State's Department of Health as Medical Director for Maternal and Child Health, he designed and then helped execute a successful mass immunization program for children in the face of a national measles epidemic. He has also worked in partnership with UNICEF to implement safe immunization practices worldwide as Worldwide Medical Director of Immunization at a large medical technology company.

Dr Rosenberg obtained his B.A. from Stanford University, earned his M.D. at the University of California, San Francisco, and completed his Residency at Cornell University Medical School. Dr Rosenberg obtained an M.P.H. in Epidemiology from Columbia University's School of Public Health. He is an elected Fellow, American College of Preventive Medicine, as well as Fellow, New York Academy of Medicine.